Keto Chaffle Recipes Cookbook Bible:

Quick and Easy mouth-watering recipes to lose weight fast, burn fat and eat well with amazing dishes

SARAH BUCKLEY

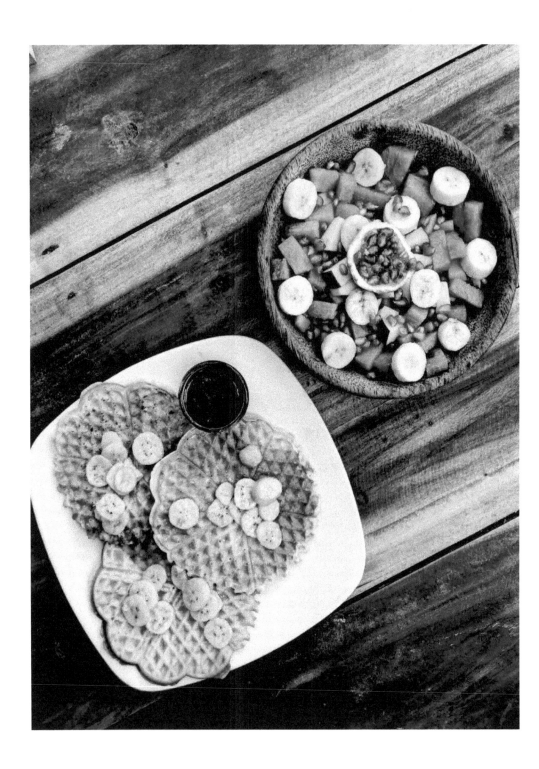

Text Copyright © [Sarah Buckley]

All rights reserved. No part of this guide may be reproduced in any form without permission in writing from the publisher except in the case of brief quotations embodied in critical articles or reviews.

Legal & Disclaimer

The information contained in this book and its contents is not designed to replace or take the place of any form of medical or professional advice; and is not meant to replace the need for independent medical, financial, legal or other professional advice or services, as may be required. The content and information in this book have been provided for educational and entertainment purposes only.

The content and information contained in this book have been compiled from sources deemed reliable, and it is accurate to the best of the Author's knowledge, information, and belief. However, the author cannot guarantee its accuracy and validity and cannot be held liable for any errors and/or omissions. Further, changes are periodically made to this book as and when needed. Where appropriate and/or necessary, you must consult a professional (including but not limited to your doctor, attorney, financial advisor or such other professional advisor) before using any of the suggested remedies, techniques, or information in this book.

Upon using the contents and information contained in this book, you agree to hold harmless the Author from and against any damages, costs, and expenses, including any legal fees potentially resulting from the application of any of the information provided by this book. This disclaimer applies to any loss, damages or injury caused by the use and application, whether directly or indirectly, of any advice or information presented, whether for breach of contract, tort, negligence, personal injury, criminal intent, or under any other cause of action.

You agree to accept all risks of using the information presented inside this book.

You agree that by continuing to read this book, where appropriate and/or necessary, you shall consult a professional (including but not limited to your doctor, attorney, or financial advisor or such other advisor as needed) before using any of the suggested remedies, techniques, or information in this book.

TABLE OF CONTENTS

TABLE OF CONTENTS 5

INTRODUCTION 9

How to Make Chaffles? 11

11 Tips to Make Chaffles 11

SIMPLE CHAFFLES 14

1. Chaffle Cannoli 14

2. Strawberry Shortcake Chaffle Bowls 16

3. Chocolate Melt Chaffles 18

4. Pumpkin & Pecan Chaffle 20

5. Spicy Jalapeno & Bacon Chaffles 22

6. Zucchini Parmesan Chaffles 24

7. Cheddar & Almond Flour Chaffles 25

8. Simple& Beginner Chaffle 26

9. Asian Cauliflower Chaffles 27

10. Sharp Cheddar Chaffles 29

BREAKFAST CHAFFLE RECIPE .30

11. Hot Ham Chaffles 30

12.	Bacon & Egg Chaffles	32
13.	Cheese-free Breakfast Chaffle	34
14.	Bacon Chaffle Omelettes	35
15.	Acocado Chaffle Toast	37
16.	Keto Chaffle Waffle	39
17.	Keto Chaffle Topped with Salted Caramel Syrup	41
18.	Keto Chaffle Bacon Sandwich	43
19.	Crispy Zucchini Chaffle	45
20.	Peanut Butter Chaffle	47

LUNCH CHAFFLE RECIPES 49

21.	Chaffle Egg Sandwich	49
22.	Chaffle Minutes Sandwich	50
23.	Chaffle Cheese Sandwich	52
24.	Chicken Zinger Chaffle	53

BASIC CHAFFLES 55

25.	Buffalo Chicken Chaffle Recipe	55
26.	Jamaican Jerk Chicken Chaffle	57
27.	Wasabi Chaffles	59
28.	Loaded Chaffle Nachos	61

29. Mozzarella Panini 63

30. Lox Bagel Chaffle 65

SWEET CHAFFLES.....................67

31. Chocolate Chips Chaffles 67

32. Cream Cake Chaffle 69

33. Almond Butter Chaffles 71

34. Layered Chaffles 72

35. Simple Mozzarella Chaffles 73

36. Cream Mini-chaffles 74

37. Raspberry Chaffles 76

38. Lemon Chaffles 78

39. Chocolate Chip Chaffles 80

40. Pumpkin & Psyllium Husk Chaffles 82

SAVORY CHAFFLES RECIPES 84

41. Simple Grilled Cheese Chaffle 84

42. Bbq Rub Chaffles 86

43. Ham Chaffles 87

44. Cheddar Jalapeño Chaffle 89

45. Taco Chaffles 91

46.   Spinach & Cauliflower Chaffles 92

47.   Rosemary Chaffles 94

48.   Zucchini Chaffles With Peanut Butter.......................95

49.   Zucchini Chaffles...97

50.   Chicken & Jalapeño Chaffles.................................99

CONCLUSION..............................101

INTRODUCTION

If you want to lose weight or need to burn fat, you can use keto chavel in your diet plan. Keto muffins are a dietary supplement and contain no calories or carbohydrates. It also contains low carbohydrates and low calories. Keto foil cakes can help reduce weight.

How it works: The foil skin consists of chopped coconut and pumpkin seeds. It works by providing a low-calorie carbohydrate source that provides energy to your body while keeping your blood sugar stable. As you continue to use metal foil, it helps suppress hunger and increase fat burning.

Foil is made from coconut and pumpkin, and it is a healthy low-carb alternative for those who want to lose weight. When used as part of a healthy diet, the metal foil helps stabilize blood sugar levels, so the body can more easily sense time when it needs food. Keto shell does not contain any calories or carbohydrates and is an ideal tool for anyone who wants to lose weight or maintain weight.

Usually, keto diet therapists will look for precise dietary methods and at the same time find ways to make life easier. I find them very easy to fix, and thankfully, they can be enjoyed at different times of the day. In the recipe below, I share a variety of ways to make and use muffins-from breakfast to dinner, snacks and desserts.

Finally, they are very convenient to eat. Moreover, we know how preparing meals can help an effective keto diet. Muffins can be frozen for later use and taste great when heated and eaten later.

Once you are obsessed with muffins, they will become a key part of your eating due to the benefits they bring. I have been making them for several weeks in a row and am considering creating a second cookbook for my newly discovered fife.

How to Make Chaffles?

Equipment and Ingredients Discussed

Making chaffles requires five simple steps and nothing more than a waffle maker for flat chaffles and a waffle bowl maker for chaffle bowls.

To make chaffles, you will need two necessary ingredients – eggs and cheese. My preferred cheeses are cheddar cheese or mozzarella cheese. These melt quickly, making them the go-to for most recipes. Meanwhile, always ensure that your cheeses are finely grated or thinly sliced for use.

Now, to make a standard chaffle:

- First, preheat your waffle maker until adequately hot.

- Meanwhile, in a bowl, mix the egg with cheese on hand until well combined.

- Open the iron, pour in a quarter or half of the mixture, and close.

- Cook the chaffle for 5 to 7 minutes or until it is crispy.

- Transfer the chaffle to a plate and allow cooling before serving.

11 Tips to Make Chaffles

My surefire ways to turn out the crispiest of chaffles:

- **Preheat Well:** Yes! It sounds obvious to preheat the waffle iron before usage. However, preheating the iron moderately will not get your chaffles as crispy as you will like. The best way to preheat before cooking is to ensure that the iron is very hot.

- **Not-So-Cheesy:** Will you prefer to have your chaffles less cheesy? Then, use mozzarella cheese.

- **Not-So Eggy**: If you aren't comfortable with the smell of eggs in your chaffles, try using egg whites instead of egg yolks or whole eggs.

- **To Shred or to Slice:** Many recipes call for shredded cheese when making chaffles, but I find sliced cheeses to offer crispier pieces. While I stick with mostly shredded cheese for convenience's sake, be at ease to use sliced cheese in the same quantity. When using sliced cheeses, arrange two to four pieces in the waffle iron, top with the beaten eggs, and some slices of the cheese. Cover and cook until crispy.

- **Shallower Irons:** For better crisps on your chaffles, use shallower waffle irons as they cook easier and faster.

- **Layering:** Don't fill up the waffle iron with too much batter. Work between a quarter and a half cup of total ingredients per batch for correctly done chaffles.

- **Patience:** It is a virtue even when making chaffles. For the best results, allow the chaffles to sit in the iron for 5 to 7 minutes before serving.

- **No Peeking:** 7 minutes isn't too much of a time to wait for the outcome of your chaffles, in my opinion. Opening the iron and checking on the chaffle before it is done stands you a worse chance of ruining it.

- **Crispy Cooling:** For better crisp, I find that allowing the chaffles to cool further after they are transferred to a plate aids a lot.

- **Easy Cleaning:** For the best cleanup, wet a paper towel and wipe the inner parts of the iron clean while still warm. Kindly note that the iron should be warm but not hot!

- **Brush It:** Also, use a clean toothbrush to clean between the iron's teeth for a thorough cleanup. You may also use a dry, rough sponge to clean the iron while it is still warm

SIMPLE CHAFFLES

1. Chaffle Cannoli

Preparation time: 9 minutes

Cooking Time: 28 Minutes

Servings: 2

Ingredients:

- For the chaffles:
- 1 large egg
- 1 egg yolk
- 3 tbsp butter, melted
- 1 tbso swerve confectioner's
- 1 cup finely grated Parmesan cheese
- 2 tbsp finely grated mozzarella cheese
- For the cannoli filling:
- ½ cup ricotta cheese
- 2 tbsp swerve confectioner's sugar
- 1 tsp vanilla extract
- 2 tbsp unsweetened chocolate chips for garnishing

Directions:

1. Preheat the waffle iron.
2. Meanwhile, in a medium bowl, mix all the ingredients for the chaffles.
3. Open the iron, pour in a quarter of the mixture, cover, and cook until crispy, 7 minutes.
4. Remove the chaffle onto a plate and make 3 more with the remaining batter.
5. Meanwhile, for the cannoli filling:
6. Beat the ricotta cheese and swerve confectioner's sugar until smooth. Mix in the vanilla.
7. On each chaffle, spread some of the filling and wrap over.
8. Garnish the creamy ends with some chocolate chips.
9. Serve immediately.

Nutrition: Calories 308Fats 25.05gCarbs 5.17gNet Carbs 5.17gProtein 15.18g

2. Strawberry Shortcake Chaffle Bowls

Preparation time: 15 minutes

Cooking Time: 28 Minutes

Servings: 2

Ingredients:

- 1 egg, beaten
- ½ cup finely grated mozzarella cheese
- 1 tbsp almond flour
- ¼ tsp baking powder
- 2 drops cake batter extract
- 1 cup cream cheese, softened
- 1 cup fresh strawberries, sliced
- 1 tbsp sugar-free maple syrup

Directions:

1. Preheat a waffle bowl maker and grease lightly with cooking spray.
2. Meanwhile, in a medium bowl, whisk all the ingredients except the cream cheese and strawberries.
3. Open the iron, pour in half of the mixture, cover, and cook until crispy, 6 to 7 minutes.

4. Remove the chaffle bowl onto a plate and set aside.

5. Make a second chaffle bowl with the remaining batter.

6. To serve, divide the cream cheese into the chaffle bowls and top with the strawberries.

7. Drizzle the filling with the maple syrup and serve.

Nutrition: Calories 235Fats 20.62gCarbs 5.9gNet Carbs 5gProtein 7.51g

3. Chocolate Melt Chaffles

Preparation time: 9 minutes

Cooking Time: 36 Minutes

Servings: 2

Ingredients:

- For the chaffles:
- 2 eggs, beaten
- ¼ cup finely grated Gruyere cheese
- 2 tbsp heavy cream
- 1 tbsp coconut flour
- 2 tbsp cream cheese, softened
- 3 tbsp unsweetened cocoa powder
- 2 tsp vanilla extract
- A pinch of salt
- For the chocolate sauce:
- 1/3 cup + 1 tbsp heavy cream
- 1 ½ oz unsweetened baking chocolate, chopped
- 1 ½ tsp sugar-free maple syrup
- 1 ½ tsp vanilla extract

Directions:

1. For the chaffles:

2. Preheat the waffle iron.

3. In a medium bowl, mix all the ingredients for the chaffles.

4. Open the iron and add a quarter of the mixture. Close and cook until crispy, 7 minutes.

5. Transfer the chaffle to a plate and make 3 more with the remaining batter.

6. For the chocolate sauce:

7. Pour the heavy cream into saucepan and simmer over low heat, 3 minutes.

8. Turn the heat off and add the chocolate. Allow melting for a few minutes and stir until fully melted, 5 minutes.

9. Mix in the maple syrup and vanilla extract.

10. Assemble the chaffles in layers with the chocolate sauce sandwiched between each layer.

11. Slice and serve immediately.

Nutrition: Calories 172Fats 13.57gCarbs 6.65gNet Carbs 3.65gProtein 5.76g

4. Pumpkin & Pecan Chaffle

Preparation time: 10 minutes

Cooking Time: 10 Minutes

Servings: 2

Ingredients:

- 1 egg, beaten
- ½ cup mozzarella cheese, grated
- ½ teaspoon pumpkin spice
- 1 tablespoon pureed pumpkin
- 2 tablespoons almond flour
- 1 teaspoon sweetener
- 2 tablespoons pecans, chopped

Directions:

1. Turn on the waffle maker.
2. Beat the egg in a bowl.
3. Stir in the rest of the ingredients.
4. Pour half of the mixture into the device.
5. Seal the lid.
6. Cook for 5 minutes.
7. Remove the chaffle carefully.
8. Repeat the steps to make the second chaffle.

Nutrition: Calories 210Total Fat 17 g Saturated Fat 10 g Cholesterol 110 mg Sodium 250 mg Potassium 570 mg Total Carbohydrate 4.6 g Dietary Fiber 1.7 g Protein 11 g Total Sugars 2 g

5. Spicy Jalapeno & Bacon Chaffles

Preparation time: 10 minutes

Servings:2

Cooking Time: 5 Minutes

Ingredients:

- 1 oz. cream cheese
- 1 large egg
- 1/2 cup cheddar cheese
- 2 tbsps. bacon bits
- 1/2 tbsp. jalapenos
- 1/4 tsp baking powder

Directions:

1. Switch on your waffle maker.
2. Grease your waffle maker with cooking spray and let it heat up.
3. Mix together egg and vanilla extract in a bowl first.
4. Add baking powder, jalapenos and bacon bites.
5. Add in cheese last and mix together.
6. Pour the chaffles batter into the maker and cook the chaffles for about 2-3 minutes
7. Once chaffles are cooked, remove from the maker.

8. Serve hot and enjoy!

Nutrition: Protein: 24% 5kcal Fat: 70% 175 kcal Carbohydrates: 6% 15 kcal

6. Zucchini Parmesan Chaffles

Preparation time: 10 minutes

Cooking Time: 14 Minutes

Servings: 2

Ingredients:

- 1 cup shredded zucchini
- 1 egg, beaten
- ½ cup finely grated Parmesan cheese
- Salt and freshly ground black pepper to taste

Directions:

1. Preheat the waffle iron.
2. Put all the ingredients in a medium bowl and mix well.
3. Open the iron and add half of the mixture. Close and cook until crispy, 7 minutes.
4. Remove the chaffle onto a plate and make another with the remaining mixture.
5. Cut each chaffle into wedges and serve afterward.

Nutrition: Calories 138Fats 9.07gCarbs 3.81gNet Carbs 3.71gProtein 10.02g

7. Cheddar & Almond Flour Chaffles

Preparation time: 10 minutes

Cooking Time: 10 Minutes

Servings: 2

Ingredients:

- 1 large organic egg, beaten
- ½ cup Cheddar cheese, shredded
- 2 tablespoons almond flour

Directions:

1. Preheat a mini waffle iron and then grease it.
2. In a bowl, place the egg, Cheddar cheese and almond flour and beat until well combined.
3. Place half of the mixture into preheated waffle iron and cook for about 5 minutes or until golden brown.
4. Repeat with the remaining mixture.
5. Serve warm.

Nutrition: Calories: 195Net Carb: 1gFat: 15.Saturated Fat: 7gCarbohydrates: 1.8gDietary Fiber: 0.8g Sugar: 0.6gProtein: 10.2g

8. Simple& Beginner Chaffle

Preparation time: 10 minutes

Servings:2

Cooking Time: 5 Minutes

Ingredients:

- 1 large egg
- 1/2 cup mozzarella cheese, shredded
- Cooking spray

Directions:

1. Switch on your waffle maker.
2. Beat the egg with a fork in a small mixing bowl.
3. Once the egg is beaten, add the mozzarella and mix well.
4. Spray the waffle maker with cooking spray.
5. Pour the chaffles mixture in a preheated waffle maker and let it cook for about 2-3 minutes.
6. Once the chaffles are cooked, carefully remove them from the maker and cook the remaining batter.
7. Serve hot with coffee and enjoy!

Nutrition: Protein: 36% 42 kcal Fat: 60% 71 kcal Carbohydrates: 4% 5 kcal

9. Asian Cauliflower Chaffles

Preparation time: 9 minutes

Cooking Time: 28 Minutes

Servings: 2

Ingredients:

- For the chaffles:
- 1 cup cauliflower rice, steamed
- 1 large egg, beaten
- Salt and freshly ground black pepper to taste
- 1 cup finely grated Parmesan cheese
- 1 tsp sesame seeds
- ¼ cup chopped fresh scallions
- For the dipping sauce:
- 3 tbsp coconut aminos
- 1 ½ tbsp plain vinegar
- 1 tsp fresh ginger puree
- 1 tsp fresh garlic paste
- 3 tbsp sesame oil
- 1 tsp fish sauce
- 1 tsp red chili flakes

Directions:

1. Preheat the waffle iron.
2. In a medium bowl, mix the cauliflower rice, egg, salt, black pepper, and Parmesan cheese.
3. Open the iron and add a quarter of the mixture. Close and cook until crispy, 7 minutes.
4. Transfer the chaffle to a plate and make 3 more chaffles in the same manner.
5. Meanwhile, make the dipping sauce.
6. In a medium bowl, mix all the ingredients for the dipping sauce.
7. Plate the chaffles, garnish with the sesame seeds and scallions and serve with the dipping sauce.

Nutrition: Calories 231Fats 188gCarbs 6.32gNet Carbs 5.42gProtein 9.66g

10. Sharp Cheddar Chaffles

Preparation time: 10 minutes

Cooking Time: 10 Minutes

Servings: 2

Ingredients:

- 1 organic egg, beaten
- ½ cup sharp Cheddar cheese, shredded

Directions:

1. Preheat a mini waffle iron and then grease it.
2. In a small bowl, place the egg and cheese and stir to combine.
3. Place half of the mixture into preheated waffle iron and cook for about 5 minutes or until golden brown.
4. Repeat with the remaining mixture.
5. Serve warm.

Nutrition: Calories: 145Net Carb: 0.5gFat: 11.Saturated Fat: 6.6gCarbohydrates: 0.5gDietary Fiber: 0g Sugar: 0.3gProtein: 9.8g

BREAKFAST CHAFFLE RECIPE

11. Hot Ham Chaffles

Preparation Time: 5 minutes

Cooking Time: 4 minutes

Servings: 4

Ingredients:

- ½ cup mozzarella cheese, shredded
- 1 egg
- ¼ cup ham, chopped
- ¼ tsp salt
- 2 tbsp mayonnaise
- 1 tsp Dijon mustard

Directions:

1. Preheat your waffle iron.
2. In the meantime, add the egg in a small mixing bowl and whisk.
3. Add in the ham, cheese, and salt. Mix to combine.

4. Scoop half the mixture using a spoon and pour into the hot waffle iron.

5. Close and cook for 4 minutes.

6. Remove the waffle and place on a large plate. Repeat the process with the remaining batter.

7. In a separate small bowl, add the mayo and mustard. Mix together until smooth.

8. Slice the waffles in quarters and use the mayo mixture as the dip.

Nutrition: Calories: 110 Cal Total Fat: 12 g Saturated Fat: 0 g Cholesterol: 0 mg Sodium: 0 mg Total Carbs: 6 g Fiber: 0 g Sugar: 0 g Protein: 12 g

12. **Bacon & Egg Chaffles**

Preparation Time: 5 minutes

Cooking Time: 10 minutes

Servings: 2

Ingredients:

- 2 eggs
- 4 tsp collagen peptides, grass-fed
- 2 tbsp pork panko
- 3 slices crispy bacon

Directions:

1. Warm up your mini waffle maker.
2. Combine the eggs, pork panko, and collagen peptides. Mix well. Divide the batter in two small bowls.
3. Once done, evenly distribute ½ of the crispy chopped bacon on the waffle maker.
4. Pour one bowl of the batter over the bacon. Cook for 5 minutes and immediately repeat this step for the second chaffle.
5. Plate your cooked chaffles and sprinkle with extra Panko for an added crunch.
6. Enjoy!

Nutrition: Calories: 266 Cal Total Fat: 17 g Saturated Fat: 0 g Cholesterol: 0 mg Sodium: 0 mg Total Carbs: 11.2 g Fiber: 0 g Sugar: 0 g Protein: 27 g

13. **Cheese-free Breakfast Chaffle**

Preparation Time: 4 minutes

Cooking Time: 12 minutes

Servings: 1

Ingredients:

- 1 egg
- ½ cup almond milk ricotta, finely shredded.
- 1 tbsp almond flour
- 2 tbsp butter

Directions:

1. Mix the egg, almond flour and ricotta in a small bowl.
2. Separate the chaffle batter into two and cook each for 4 minutes.
3. Melt the butter and pour on top of the chaffles.
4. Put them back in the pan and cook on each side for 2 minutes.
5. Remove from the pan and allow them sit for 2 minutes.
6. Enjoy while still crispy.

Nutrition: Calories: 530 Cal Total Fat: 50 g Saturated Fat: 0 g Cholesterol: 0 mg Sodium: 0 mg Total Carbs: 3 g Fiber: 0 g Sugar: 0 g Protein: 23 g

14. **Bacon Chaffle Omelettes**

Preparation Time: 5 minutes

Cooking Time: 10 minutes

Servings: 2

Ingredients:

- 2 slices bacon, raw
- 1 egg
- 1 tsp maple extract, optional
- 1 tsp all spices

Directions:

1. Put the bacon slices in a blender and turn it on.
2. Once ground up, add in the egg and all spices. Go on blending until liquefied.
3. Heat your waffle maker on the highest setting and spray with non-stick cooking spray.
4. Pour half the omelette into the waffle maker and cook for 5 minutes max.
5. Remove the crispy omelette and repeat the same steps with rest batter.
6. Enjoy warm.

Nutrition: Calories: 59 Cal Total Fat: 4.4 g Saturated Fat: 0 g Cholesterol: 0 mg Sodium: 0 mg Total Carbs: 1 g Fiber: 0 g Sugar: 0 g Protein: 5 g

15. <u>Acocado Chaffle Toast</u>

Preparation Time: 4 minutes

Cooking Time: 8 minutes

Servings: 2

Ingredients:

- ½ avocado
- 1 egg
- ½ cup cheddar cheese, finely shredded
- 1 tbsp almond flour
- 1 tsp lemon juice, fresh
- Salt, ground pepper to taste
- Parmesan cheese, finely shredded for garnishing

Directions:

1. Warm up your mini waffle maker.
2. Mix the egg, almond flour with cheese in a small bowl.
3. For a crispy crust, add a teaspoon of shredded cheese to the waffle maker and cook for 30 seconds.
4. Then, pour the mixture into the waffle maker and cook for 5 minutes or until crispy.
5. Repeat with remaining batter.

6. Mash avocado with a fork until well combined and add lemon juice, salt, pepper

7. Top each chaffle with avocado mixture. Sprinkle with parmesan and enjoy!

Nutrition: Calories: 250 Cal Total Fat: 23 g Saturated Fat: 0 g Cholesterol: 0 mg Sodium: 0 mg Total Carbs: 9 g Fiber: 0 g Sugar: 0 g Protein: 14 g

16. **Keto Chaffle Waffle**

Preparation time:

Cooking time:

Ingredients:

- 1 egg
- ½ cup of shredded mozzarella cheese
- 1 ½ table-spoon of almond flour
- Pinch of baking powder
- Equipment:
- Waffle Maker
- Shredder (to shred solid mozzarella cheese)

Directions:

1. Start by turning your waffle maker on and preheating it. During the time of pre-heating, in a bowl, whisk the egg and shredded mozzarella cheese together. If you do not have shredded mozzarella cheese, you can use the shredder to shred your cheese, then add the almond powder and baking powder to the bowl and whisk them until the mixture is consistent.

2. Then pour the mixture onto the waffle machine. Make sure you pour it to the center of the mixture will come

out of the edges on closing the machine. Close the machine and let the waffles cook until golden brown. Then you can serve your tasty chaffle waffles.

Nutrition: Serves 1 person Calories 320 Carbohydrates 2.9 g Protein 21.5 g Fat 24.3g

17. Keto Chaffle Topped with Salted Caramel Syrup

Preparation time: 15 mins

Cooking time: 10 mins

Ingredients:

- 1 egg
- ½ cup of mozzarella cheese
- ¼ cup of cream
- 2 tablespoon of collagen powder
- 1 ½ tablespoon of almond flour
- 1 ½ tablespoon of unsalted butter
- Pinch of salt
- ¾ tablespoon of powdered erythritol
- Pinch of baking powder

Directions:

1. Begin by preheating your waffle machine by switching it on and turning the heat to medium. Whisk together the chaffle ingredients that include the egg, mozzarella cheese, almond flour, and baking powder. Pour the mixture on the waffle machine. Let it cook until golden

brown. You can make up to two chaffles with this method.

2. To make the caramel syrup, you will need to turn on the flame under a pan to medium heat Melt the unsalted butter on the pan. Then turn the heat low and add collagen powder and erythritol to the pan and whisk them. Gradually add the cream and remove from heat. Then add the salt and continue to whisk. Pour the syrup onto the chaffle, and here you go.

Nutrition: 1 serving 605 calories 45g fat 48g protein 5.1 g of carbohydrates

18. **Keto Chaffle Bacon Sandwich**

Preparation time: 15 mins

Cooking time: 10 mins

Ingredients:

- 1 egg
- ½ cup of shredded mozzarella cheese
- 2 Tablespoon of coconut flour
- 2 strips of pork or beef bacon
- 1 slice of any type of cheese
- 2 tablespoon of coconut oil

Directions:

1. To make the chaffle, you will be following the typical recipe for making a chaffle. Start by warming your waffle machine to medium heat. In a bowl, beat 1 egg, ½ cup of mozzarella cheese, and almond flour. Pour the mixture on the waffle machine. Let it cook until it is golden brown. Then remove in a plate.

2. Warm coconut oil in a pan over medium heat. Then place the bacon strips in the pan. Cook until crispy over medium heat. Assemble the bacon and cheese on the chaffle.

Nutrition: Serving size 1 Calories 580 Fat 52 g Carbohydrates 3g

19. Crispy Zucchini Chaffle

Preparation time: 15 mins

Cooking time: 5 mins

Ingredients:

- 2 eggs
- 1 fresh zucchini
- 1 cup of shredded or grated cheddar cheese
- 2 pinch of salt
- 1 tablespoon of onion (chopped)
- 1 clove of garlic

Directions:

1. Start by preheating the waffle maker to medium heat. The best way to make a chaffle is to make it with layering. Start by dicing onions and mashing the garlic. Then use the grater to grate the zucchini. Then take a bowl and add 2 eggs and add the grated zucchini to the bowl.

2. Also, add the onions, salt, and garlic for extra flavor. You can also add other herbs to give your zaffle a crispy more flavor. Then sprinkle ½ cup of cheese on top of the waffle machine.

3. Add the mixture from the bowl to the waffle machine. Add the remaining cheese on top of the waffle machine and close the waffle machine. Make sure the waffle cooks for about 3 to 5 minutes until it turns golden brown.

4. By the layering method, you will achieve the perfect crisp. Take out your zucchini chaffles and serve them hot and fresh.

5. Equipment:

6. Waffle maker

7. Grater to grate the cheese

Nutrition: Serving size 2 Calories 170 Fat 12g Carbohydrates 4g Protein 11g

20. Peanut Butter Chaffle

Preparation time: 15 min

Cooking time: 10 min

Ingredients:

- 1 egg
- ½ cup of cheddar cheese
- 2 tablespoon of peanut butter
- Few drops of vanilla extract

Directions:

1. To make deliciously tasting peanut butter chaffles. Take a grater and grate some cheddar cheese. Add one egg, cheddar cheese, 2 tablespoon of peanut butter, and a few drops of vanilla extract. Beat these ingredients together until the batter is consistent enough.

2. Then sprinkle some shredded cheese as a base on the waffle maker. Pour the mixture on top of the waffle machine.

3. Sprinkle more cheese on top of the mixture and close the waffle machine. Ensure that the waffle is cooked thoroughly for about a few minutes until they are golden brown. Then remove it and enjoy your deliciously cooked chaffles.

4. Equipment:

5. Waffle maker

6. Grater

Nutrition: 1 serving 363 Calories 29 g of Fat 22 g of Protein 4 g of Carbohydrates

LUNCH CHAFFLE RECIPES

21. Chaffle Egg Sandwich

Preparation time: 10 minutes

Cooking Time: 10 Minutes

Servings:2

Ingredients:

- 2 minutes keto chaffle
- 2 slice cheddar cheese
- 1 egg simple omelet

Directions:

1. Prepare your oven on 4000 F.
2. Arrange egg omelet and cheese slice between chaffles.
3. Bake in the preheated oven for about 4-5 minutes Utes until cheese is melted.
4. Once the cheese is melted, remove from the oven.
5. Serve and enjoy!

Nutrition: Protein: 29% 144 kcal Fat: % 337 kcal Carbohydrates: 3% 14 kcal

22. Chaffle Minutes Sandwich

Preparation time: 10 minutes

Cooking Time: 10 Minutes

Servings:2

Ingredients:

- 1 large egg
- 1/8 cup almond flour
- 1/2 tsp. garlic powder
- 3/4 tsp. baking powder
- 1/2 cup shredded cheese
- SANDWICH FILLING
- 2 slices deli ham
- 2 slices tomatoes
- 1 slice cheddar cheese

Directions:

1. Grease your square waffle maker and preheat it on medium heat.
2. Mix together chaffle ingredients in a mixing bowl until well combined.
3. Pour batter into a square waffle and make two chaffles.
4. Once chaffles are cooked, remove from the maker.

5. For a sandwich, arrange deli ham, tomato slice and cheddar cheese between two chaffles.

6. Cut sandwich from the center.

7. Serve and enjoy!

Nutrition: Protein: 29% 70 kcal Fat: 66% 159 kcal Carbohydrates: 4% 10 kcal

23. Chaffle Cheese Sandwich

Preparation time: 10 minutes

Servings: 1

Cooking Time: 10 Minutes

Ingredients:

- 2 square keto chaffle
- 2 slice cheddar cheese
- 2 lettuce leaves

Directions:

1. Prepare your oven on 4000 F.
2. Arrange lettuce leave and cheese slice between chaffles.
3. Bake in the preheated oven for about 4-5 minutes Utes until cheese is melted.
4. Once the cheese is melted, remove from the oven.
5. Serve and enjoy!

Nutrition: Protein: 28% kcal Fat: 69% 149 kcal Carbohydrates: 3% 6 kcal

24. Chicken Zinger Chaffle

Preparation time: 10 minutes

Servings:2

Cooking Time: 15 Minutes

Ingredients:

- 1 chicken breast, cut into 2 pieces
- 1/2 cup coconut flour
- 1/4 cup finely grated Parmesan
- 1 tsp. paprika
- 1/2 tsp. garlic powder
- 1/2 tsp. onion powder
- 1 tsp. salt& pepper
- 1 egg beaten
- Avocado oil for frying
- Lettuce leaves
- BBQ sauce
- CHAFFLE Ingredients:
- 4 oz. cheese
- 2 whole eggs
- 2 oz. almond flour
- 1/4 cup almond flour

- 1 tsp baking powder

Directions:

1. Mix together chaffle ingredients in a bowl.
2. Pour the chaffle batter in preheated greased square chaffle maker.
3. Cook chaffles for about 2-minutesutes until cooked through.
4. Make square chaffles from this batter.
5. Meanwhile mix together coconut flour, parmesan, paprika, garlic powder, onion powder salt and pepper in a bowl.
6. Dip chicken first in coconut flour mixture then in beaten egg.
7. Heat avocado oil in a skillet and cook chicken from both sides. until lightly brown and cooked
8. Set chicken zinger between two chaffles with lettuce and BBQ sauce.
9. Enjoy!

Nutrition: Protein: 30% 219 kcal Fat: 60% 435 kcal Carbohydrates: 9% 66 kcal

BASIC CHAFFLES

25. Buffalo Chicken Chaffle Recipe

Preparation time: 10 minutes

Cooking time: 5 minutes

Servings: 6

Ingredients:

- 1 Can Valley Fresh Organic Canned Chicken Breast (5 ounces)
- 2 T Red Hot Wing Sauce
- 2 oz Cream Cheese softened
- 4 T Cheddar Cheese shredded
- 2 T Almond Flour
- 1 T Nutritional Yeast
- 1/2 tsp Baking Powder
- 1 Egg Yolk Can Use whole egg if no allergy
- 1 Flax Egg 1 T ground flaxseed, 3 T water
- 1/4-1/2 Cup Extra Cheese for the waffle iron

Directions:

1. Make flax egg and set aside to rest.

2. Drain liquid from the canned chicken. Mix all the ingredients together. Sprinkle a little cheese on the waffle iron. Let it sit for a few seconds before adding 3 T of chicken mixture — Cook for 5 minutes.

3. Don't open the waffle iron before the time is up, or you will have a mess. Remove and let cool before adding a drizzle of hot sauce and ranch dressing.

Nutrition: Calories 320 Carbohydrates 2.9 g Protein 21.5 g Fat 24.3g

26. **Jamaican Jerk Chicken Chaffle**

Preparation time: 5 minutes

Cooking time: 10 minutes

Servings: 4

Ingredients:

- Jamaican Jerk Chicken Filling:
- 1 pound organic ground chicken browned or roasted leftover chicken finely chopped
- 2 tablespoons Kerrygold butter
- 1/2 medium onion chopped
- 1 teaspoon granulated garlic
- 1 teaspoon dried thyme
- 1/8 teaspoon black pepper
- 2 teaspoon dried parsley
- 1 teaspoon salt
- 2 teaspoon Walker's Wood Jerk Seasoning Hot and Spicy jar type paste
- 1/2 cup chicken broth
- Chaffle Ingredients:
- 1/2 cup mozzarella cheese
- 1 tablespoon butter melted

- 1 egg well beaten
- 2 tablespoon almond flour
- 1/4 teaspoon baking powder
- 1/4 teaspoon turmeric
- A pinch of xanthan gum
- A pinch of salt
- A pinch of garlic powder
- A pinch of onion powder

Directions:

1. In a medium saucepan, cook onion in the butter.
2. Add all spices and herbs. Sauté until fragrant.
3. Add chicken.
4. Stir in chicken broth.
5. Cook on low for 10 minutes.
6. Raise temperature to medium-high and reduce liquid until none is left in the bottom of the pan.
7. Enjoy!

Nutrition: Calories 320 Carbohydrates 2.9 g Protein 21.5 g Fat 24.3g

27. <u>Wasabi Chaffles</u>

Preparation time: 15 minutes

Cooking time: 15 minutes

Servings: 1

Chaffle Ingredients:

- Classic Chaffle Recipe
- Japanese Toppings Ingredients:
- 1 whole avocado, ripe
- 5 slices of pickled ginger
- 1 tbsp of gluten-free soy sauce
- 1/3 of a cup of edamame
- 1/4 of a cup of Japanese pickled vegetables
- 1/2 pound of sushi-grade salmon, sliced
- 1/4 of a tsp of wasabi
- Tools: waffle maker, mini or regular sized, one mixing bowl, measuring cups and tablespoons, spatula, non-stick cooking spray (or butter), blender, electric beaters, or whisk.

Directions:

1. Cut the salmon and avocado into thin slices. Set aside.

2. If the edamame is frozen, boil it in a pot of water until done. Set aside.

3. Follow the Classic Chaffle recipe.

4. Once the chaffles are done, pour a tablespoon of soy sauce onto the chaffle and then layer the salmon, avocado, edamame, pickled ginger, pickled vegetables, and wasabi.

5. Enjoy!

Nutrition: Calories 320 Carbohydrates 2.9 g Protein 21.5 g Fat 24.3g

28. **Loaded Chaffle Nachos**

Preparation time: 15 minutes

Cooking time: 15 minutes

Servings: 1

Chaffle Ingredients:

- Classic Chaffle Recipe
- Nacho Ingredients:
- Taco Meat recipe
- 1 whole avocado, ripe
- 1/2 cup of sour cream
- 1/2 of a cup of cheddar cheese, shredded
- 1/2 an onion
- 1 handful of cilantro, chopped
- 1 lime, cut into wedges
- hot sauce of your choice
- Tools: waffle maker, mini or regular sized, one mixing bowl, measuring cups and tablespoons, spatula, non-stick cooking spray (or butter), blender, electric beaters, or whisk.

Directions:

1. Dice the cilantro, lettuce, onions, and limes.

2. Shred the cheese in a bowl. Melt if desired.

3. Follow instructions for the Taco Meat recipe.

4. Follow the Classic Chaffle recipe.

5. Once the chaffles are done, rip them into triangles.

6. Spread the chaffle triangles onto a plate and layer on the sour cream, meat, avocado, onions, cilantro, cheese, and lime.

7. Enjoy!

Nutrition: Calories 320 Carbohydrates 2.9 g Protein 21.5 g Fat 24.3g

29. Mozzarella Panini

Preparation time: 15 minutes

Cooking time: 15 minutes

Servings: 1

Chaffle Ingredients:

- Classic Chaffle Recipe
- Sandwich Filling Ingredients:
- 1 ounce of mozzarella, thinly sliced
- 1 heirloom tomato, thinly sliced
- 1/4 of a cup of pesto
- 2 fresh basil leaves
- Tools: waffle maker, mini or regular sized, one mixing bowl, measuring cups and tablespoons, spatula, non-stick cooking spray (or butter), blender, electric beaters, or whisk.

Directions:

1. Follow the Classic Chaffle recipe.
2. Once the chaffles are done, lay two side by side.
3. Spread the pesto on one, then layer the mozzarella cheese and tomatoes and sandwich together.

Nutrition: Calories 320 Carbohydrates 2.9 g Protein 21.5 g Fat 24.3g

30. Lox Bagel Chaffle

Preparation time: 15 minutes

Cooking time: 15 minutes

Servings: 1

Chaffle Ingredients:

- Classic Chaffle Recipe or Sweet Chaffle Recipe
- 2 tbsps of Everything Bagel Seasoning
- Filling Ingredients:
- 1 ounce of cream cheese
- 1 beefsteak tomato, thinly sliced
- 4-6 ounces of salmon gravlax
- 1 small shallot, thinly sliced
- capers
- 1 tbsp of fresh dill
- Tools: waffle maker, mini or regular sized, one mixing bowl, measuring cups and tablespoons, spatula, non-stick cooking spray (or butter), blender, electric beaters, or whisk.

Directions:

1. Slice the tomato and the shallots.

2. Follow the Classic Chaffle recipe and add the everything bagel seasoning.
3. Once the chaffles are done, sprinkle more everything bagel seasoning onto the tops of both chaffles.
4. Lay two chaffles side by side and layer on the cream cheese, salmon, and shallots.
5. Sprinkle dill and capers and sandwich the two chaffles together.
6. Enjoy!

Nutrition: Calories 320 Carbohydrates 2.9 g Protein 21.5 g Fat 24.3g

SWEET CHAFFLES

31. Chocolate Chips Chaffles

Preparation time: 5 minutes

Cooking Time: 8 Minutes

Servings: 2

Ingredients:

- 1 large organic egg
- 1 teaspoon coconut flour
- 1 teaspoon Erythritol
- ½ teaspoon organic vanilla extract
- ½ cup Mozzarella cheese, shredded finely
- 2 tablespoons 70% dark chocolate chips

Directions:

1. Preheat a mini waffle iron and then grease it.
2. In a bowl, place the egg, coconut flour, sweetener and vanilla extract and beat until well combined.
3. Add the cheese and stir to combine.
4. Place half of the mixture into preheated waffle iron and top with half of the chocolate chips.
5. Place a little egg mixture over each chocolate chip.

6. Cook for about 3-4 minutes or until golden brown.

7. Repeat with the remaining mixture and chocolate chips.

8. Serve warm.

Nutrition: Calories: 164Net Carb: 2.Fat: 11.9gSaturated Fat: 6.6gCarbohydrates: 5.4gDietary Fiber: 2.5g Sugar: 0.3gProtein: 7.3g

32. Cream Cake Chaffle

Preparation time: 8 minutes

Cooking Time: 12 Minutes

Servings: 2

Ingredients:

- Chaffle
- 4 oz cream cheese, softened
- 4 eggs
- 4 tbsp coconut flour
- 1 tbsp almond flour
- 1 ½ tsp baking powder
- 1 tbsp butter, softened
- 1 tsp vanilla extract
- ½ tsp cinnamon
- 1 tbsp sweetener
- 1 tbsp shredded coconut, colored and unsweetened
- 1 tbsp walnuts, chopped
- Italian Cream Frosting
- 2 oz cream cheese, softened
- 2 tbsp butter, room temperature
- 2 tbsp sweetener

- ½ tsp vanilla

Directions:

1. Preheat your waffle maker and add ¼ of the
2. Cook for 3 minutes and repeat the process until you have 4 chaffles.
3. Remove and set aside.
4. In the meantime, start making your frosting by mixing all the
5. Stir until you have a smooth and creamy mixture.
6. Cool, frost the cake and enjoy.

Nutrition: Calories per Servings: 127 Kcal ; Fats: 10 g ;

Carbs: 5.5 g ; Protein: 7 g

33. **Almond Butter Chaffles**

Preparation time: 5 minutes

Cooking Time: 10 Minutes

Servings: 2

Ingredients:

- 1 large organic egg, beaten
- 1/3 cup Mozzarella cheese, shredded
- 1 tablespoon Erythritol
- 2 tablespoons almond butter
- 1 teaspoon organic vanilla extract

Directions:

1. Preheat a mini waffle iron and then grease it.
2. In a medium bowl, place all ingredients and with a fork, mix until well combined.
3. Place half of the mixture into preheated waffle iron and cook for about 5 minutes or until golden brown.
4. Repeat with the remaining mixture.
5. Serve warm.

Nutrition: Calories: 153Net Carb: 2gFat: 12.3gSaturated Fat: 2gCarbohydrates: 3.Dietary Fiber: 1.6g Sugar: 1.2gProtein: 7.9g

34. Layered Chaffles

Preparation time: 5 minutes

Cooking Time: 10 Minutes

Servings: 2

Ingredients:

- 1 organic egg, beaten and divided
- ½ cup cheddar cheese, shredded and divided
- Pinch of salt

Directions:

1. Preheat a mini waffle iron and then grease it.
2. Place about 1/8 cup of cheese in the bottom of the waffle iron and top with half of the beaten egg.
3. Now, place 1/8 cup of cheese on top and cook for about 4–5 minutes.
4. Repeat with the remaining cheese and egg.
5. Serve warm.

Nutrition: Calories 145 Net Carbs 0.5 g Total Fat 11.g Saturated Fat 6.6 g Cholesterol 112 mg Sodium 284 g Total Carbs 0.5 g Fiber 0 g Sugar 0.3 g Protein 9.8 g

35. Simple Mozzarella Chaffles

Preparation time: 5 minutes

Cooking Time: 8 Minutes

Servings: 2

Ingredients:

- ½ cup mozzarella cheese, shredded
- 1 large organic egg
- 2 tablespoons blanched almond flour
- ¼ teaspoon organic baking powder
- 2–3 drops liquid stevia

Directions:

1. Preheat a mini waffle iron and then grease it.
2. In a medium bowl, put all ingredients and with a fork, mix until well combined. Place half of the mixture into preheated waffle iron and cook for about 3–4 minutes.
3. Repeat with the remaining mixture.
4. Serve warm.

Nutrition: Calories 98 Net Carbs 1.4 g Total Fat 7.1 g Saturated Fat 1.8 g Cholesterol 97 mg Sodium 81 mg Total Carbs 2.2 g Fiber 0.8 g Sugar 0.2 g Protein 6.7 g

36. Cream Mini-chaffles

Preparation time: 5 minutes

Cooking Time: 10 Minutes

Servings: 2

Ingredients:

- 2 tsp coconut flour
- 4 tsp swerve/monk fruit
- ¼ tsp baking powder
- 1 egg
- 1 oz cream cheese
- ½ tsp vanilla extract

Directions:

1. Turn on waffle maker to heat and oil it with cooking spray.
2. Mix swerve/monk fruit, coconut flour, and baking powder in a small mixing bowl.
3. Add cream cheese, egg, vanilla extract, and whisk until well-combined.
4. Add batter into waffle maker and cook for 3-minutes, until golden brown.
5. Serve with your favorite toppings.

Nutrition: Carbs: 4 g ;Fat: g ;Protein: 2 g ;Calories: 73

37. **Raspberry Chaffles**

Preparation time: 5 minutes

Cooking Time: 5 Minutes

Servings: 5

Ingredients:

- 4 Tbsp almond flour
- 4 large eggs
- 2⅓ cup shredded mozzarella cheese
- 1 tsp vanilla extract
- 1 Tbsp erythritol sweetener
- 1½ tsp baking powder
- ½ cup raspberries

Directions:

1. Turn on waffle maker to heat and oil it with cooking spray.
2. Mix almond flour, sweetener, and baking powder in a bowl.
3. Add cheese, eggs, and vanilla extract, and mix until well-combined.
4. Add 1 portion of batter to waffle maker and spread it evenly. Close and cook for 3-minutes, or until golden.

5. Repeat until remaining batter is used.

6. Serve with raspberries.

Nutrition: Carbs: 5 g ;Fat: 11 g ;Protein: 24 g ;Calories: 300

38. Lemon Chaffles

Preparation time: 5 minutes

Cooking Time: 10 Minutes

Servings: 2

Ingredients:

- 1 organic egg, beaten
- 1 ounce cream cheese, softened
- 2 tablespoons almond flour
- 1 tablespoon fresh lemon juice
- 2 teaspoons Erythritol
- ½ teaspoon fresh lemon zest, grated
- ¼ teaspoon organic baking powder
- Pinch of salt
- ½ teaspoon powdered Erythritol

Directions:

1. Preheat a mini waffle iron and then grease it.
2. In a bowl, place all ingredients except the powdered Erythritol and beat until well combined.
3. Place half of the mixture into preheated waffle iron and cook for about 5 minutes or until golden brown.
4. Repeat with the remaining mixture.

5. Serve warm with the sprinkling of powdered Erythritol.

Nutrition: Calories: 129Net Carb: 1.2gFat: 10.9gSaturated Fat: 4.1gCarbohydrates: 2.4gDietary Fiber: 0.8g Sugar: 0.Protein: 3.9g

39. Chocolate Chip Chaffles

Preparation time: 8 minutes

Servings: 1

Cooking Time: 6 Minutes

Ingredients:

- 1 egg
- 1 tsp coconut flour
- 1 tsp sweetener
- ½ tsp vanilla extract
- ¼ cup heavy whipping cream, for serving
- ½ cup almond milk ricotta, finely shredded
- 2 tbsp sugar-free chocolate chips

Directions:

1. Preheat your mini waffle iron.
2. Mix the egg, coconut flour, vanilla, and sweetener. Whisk together with a fork.
3. Stir in the almond milk ricotta.
4. Pour half of the batter into the waffle iron and dot with a pinch of chocolate chips.
5. Close the waffle iron and cook for minutes.
6. Repeat with remaining batter.

7. Serve hot with the whipped cream.

Nutrition: Calories per Servings: 304 Kcal ; Fats: 16 g ;

Carbs: 7 g ; Protein: 3 g

40. **Pumpkin & Psyllium Husk Chaffles**

Preparation time: 8 minutes

Cooking Time: 16 Minutes

Servings: 2

Ingredients:

- 2 organic eggs
- ½ cup mozzarella cheese, shredded
- 1 tablespoon homemade pumpkin puree
- 2 teaspoons Erythritol
- ½ teaspoon psyllium husk powder
- 1/3 teaspoon ground cinnamon
- Pinch of salt
- ½ teaspoon organic vanilla extract

Directions:

1. Preheat a mini waffle iron and then grease it.
2. In a bowl, place all ingredients and beat until well combined.
3. Place ¼ of the mixture into preheated waffle iron and cook for about 4 minutes or until golden brown.
4. Repeat with the remaining mixture.
5. Serve warm.

Nutrition: Calories: 4et Carb: 0.6gFat: 2.8gSaturated Fat: 1.1gCarbohydrates: 0.8gDietary Fiber: 0.2g Sugar: 0.4gProtein: 3.9g

SAVORY CHAFFLES RECIPES

41. Simple Grilled Cheese Chaffle

Preparation time: 5 minutes

Cooking Time: 10 Minutes

Servings: 2

Ingredients:

- 1 large egg
- ½ cup mozzarella cheese
- 2 slices yellow American cheese
- 2-3 slices cooked bacon, cut in half
- 1 tsp butter
- ½ tsp baking powder

Directions:

1. Turn on waffle maker to heat and oil it with cooking spray.
2. Beat egg in a bowl.
3. Add mozzarella, and baking powder.

4. Pour half of the mix into the waffle maker and cook for minutes.

5. Remove and repeat to make the second chaffle.

6. Layer bacon and cheese slices in between two chaffles.

7. Melt butter in a skillet and add chaffle sandwich to the pan. Fry on each side for 2-3 minutes covered, until cheese has melted.

8. Slice in half on a plate and serve.

Nutrition: Carbs: 4 g ;Fat: 18 g ;Protein: 7 g ;Calories: 233

42. Bbq Rub Chaffles

Preparation time: 10 minutes

Cooking Time: 20 Minutes

Servings: 2

Ingredients:

- 2 organic eggs, beaten
- 1 cup Cheddar cheese, shredded
- ½ teaspoon BBQ rub
- ¼ teaspoon organic baking powder

Directions:

1. Preheat a mini waffle iron and then grease it.
2. In a medium bowl, place all ingredients and with a fork, mix until well combined.
3. Place ¼ of the mixture into preheated waffle iron and cook for about 5 minutes or until golden brown.
4. Repeat with the remaining mixture.
5. Serve warm.

Nutrition: Calories: 14et Carb: 0.7gFat: 11.6gSaturated Fat: 6.6gCarbohydrates: 0.7gDietary Fiber: 0g Sugar: 0.3gProtein: 9.8g

43. **Ham Chaffles**

Preparation time: 10 minutes

Cooking Time: 16 Minutes

Servings: 2

Ingredients:

- 2 large organic eggs (yolks and whites separated)
- 6 tablespoons butter, melted
- 2 scoops unflavored whey protein powder
- 1 teaspoon organic baking powder
- Salt, to taste
- 1 ounce sugar-free ham, chopped finely
- 1 ounce Cheddar cheese, shredded
- 1/8 teaspoon paprika

Directions:

1. Preheat a waffle iron and then grease it.
2. In a bowl place egg yolks, butter, protein powder, baking powder and salt and beat until well combined.
3. Add the ham steak pieces, cheese and paprika and stir to combine.

4. In another bowl, place 2 egg whites and a pinch of salt and with an electric hand mixer and beat until stiff peaks form.
5. Gently fold the whipped egg whites into the egg yolk mixture in 2 batches.
6. Place ¼ of the mixture into preheated waffle iron and cook for about 3-4 minutes or until golden brown.
7. Repeat with the remaining mixture.
8. Serve warm.

Nutrition: Calories: 288Net Carb: 1.5gFat: 22.8gSaturated Fat: 13.4gCarbohydrates: 1.7gDietary Fiber: 0.2g Sugar: 0.3gProtein: 20.3g

44. Cheddar Jalapeño Chaffle

Preparation time: 6 minutes

Cooking Time: 5 Minutes

Servings: 2

Ingredients:

- 2 large eggs
- ½ cup shredded mozzarella
- ¼ cup almond flour
- ½ tsp baking powder
- ¼ cup shredded cheddar cheese
- 2 Tbsp diced jalapeños jarred or canned
- For the toppings:
- ½ cooked bacon, chopped
- 2 Tbsp cream cheese
- ¼ jalapeño slices

Directions:

1. Turn on waffle maker to heat and oil it with cooking spray.
2. Mix mozzarella, eggs, baking powder, almond flour, and garlic powder in a bowl.

3. Sprinkle 2 Tbsp cheddar cheese in a thin layer on waffle maker, and ½ jalapeño.

4. Ladle half of the egg mixture on top of the cheese and jalapeños.

5. Cook for minutes, or until done.

6. Repeat for the second chaffle.

7. Top with cream cheese, bacon, and jalapeño slices.

Nutrition: Carbs: 5 g ;Fat: 1g ;Protein: 18 g ;Calories: 307

45. Taco Chaffles

Preparation time: 10 minutes

Cooking Time: 20 Minutes

Servings: 2

Ingredients:

- 1 tablespoon almond flour
- 1 cup taco blend cheese
- 2 organic eggs
- ¼ teaspoon taco seasoning

Directions:

1. Preheat a mini waffle iron and then grease it.
2. In a bowl, place all ingredients and mix until well combined.
3. Place ¼ of the mixture into preheated waffle iron and cook for about 4 minutes or until golden brown.
4. Repeat with the remaining mixture.
5. Serve warm.

Nutrition: Calories: 71Net Carb: 0.7gFat: 5.4gSaturated Fat: 2.2gCarbohydrates: 0.9gDietary Fiber: 0.2g Sugar: 0.3gProtein: 4.5g

46. Spinach & Cauliflower Chaffles

Preparation time: 6 minutes

Cooking Time: 10 Minutes

Servings: 2

Ingredients:

- ½ cup frozen chopped spinach, thawed and squeezed
- ½ cup cauliflower, chopped finely
- ½ cup Cheddar cheese, shredded
- ½ cup Mozzarella cheese, shredded
- 1/3 cup Parmesan cheese, , shredded
- 2 organic eggs
- 1 tablespoon butter, melted
- 1 teaspoon garlic powder
- 1 teaspoon onion powder
- Salt and freshly ground black pepper, to taste

Directions:

1. Preheat a waffle iron and then grease it.
2. In a medium bowl, place all ingredients and, mix until well combined.
3. Place half of the mixture into preheated waffle iron and cook for about 4-5 minutes or until golden brown.

4. Repeat with the remaining mixture.

5. Serve warm.

Nutrition: Calories: 320Net Carb: 4gFat: 24.5gSaturated Fat: 14gCarbohydrates: 5gDietary Fiber: 1g Sugar: 1.9gProtein: 20.8g

47. Rosemary Chaffles

Preparation time: 6 minutes

Cooking Time: 8 Minutes

Servings: 2

Ingredients:

- 1 organic egg, beaten
- ½ cup Cheddar cheese, shredded
- 1 tablespoon almond flour
- 1 tablespoon fresh rosemary, chopped
- Pinch of salt and freshly ground black pepper

Directions:

1. Preheat a mini waffle iron and then grease it.
2. For chaffles: In a medium bowl, place all ingredients and with a fork, mix until well combined.
3. Place half of the mixture into preheated waffle iron and cook for about 4 minutes or until golden brown.
4. Repeat with the remaining mixture.
5. Serve warm.

Nutrition: Calories: 173Net Carb: 1.1gFat: 13.7gSaturated Fat: 9gCarbohydrates: 2.2gDietary Fiber: 1.1g Sugar: 0.4gProtein: 9.9g

48. Zucchini Chaffles With Peanut Butter

Servings:2

Cooking Time: 5 Minutes

Ingredients:

- 1 cup zucchini grated
- 1 egg beaten
- 1/2 cup shredded parmesan cheese
- 1/4 cup shredded mozzarella cheese
- 1 tsp dried basil
- 1/2 tsp. salt
- 1/2 tsp. black pepper
- 2 tbsps. peanut butter for topping

Directions:

1. Sprinkle salt over zucchini and let it sit for minutes Utes.
2. Squeeze out water from zucchini.
3. Beat egg with zucchini, basil. salt mozzarella cheese, and pepper.

4. Sprinkle ½ of the parmesan cheese over preheated waffle maker and pour zucchini batter over it.

5. Sprinkle the remaining cheese over it.

6. Close the lid.

7. Cook zucchini chaffles for about 4-8 minutes Utes.

8. Remove chaffles from the maker and repeat with the remaining batter.

9. Serve with peanut butter on top and enjoy!

Nutrition: Protein: 52% 88 kcal Fat: 41% 69 kcal Carbohydrates: 7% 12 kcal

49. Zucchini Chaffles

Preparation time: 10 minutes

Cooking Time: 18 Minutes

Servings: 2

Ingredients:

- 2 large zucchinis, grated and squeezed
- 2 large organic eggs
- 2/3 cup Cheddar cheese, shredded
- 2 tablespoons coconut flour
- ½ teaspoon garlic powder
- ½ teaspoon red pepper flakes, crushed
- Salt, to taste

Directions:

1. Preheat a waffle iron and then grease it.
2. In a medium bowl, place all ingredients and, mix until well combined.
3. Place ¼ of the mixture into preheated waffle iron and cook for about 4-4½ minutes or until golden brown.
4. Repeat with the remaining mixture.
5. Serve warm.

Nutrition: Calories: 159Net Carb: 4.3gFat: 10gSaturated Fat: 5.8gCarbohydrates: 8gDietary Fiber: 3.7g Sugar: 2.Protein: 10.1g

50. Chicken & Jalapeño Chaffles

Preparation time: 6 minutes

Cooking Time: 10 Minutes

Servings: 2

Ingredients:

- ½ cup grass-fed cooked chicken, chopped
- 1 organic egg, beaten
- ¼ cup Cheddar cheese, shredded
- 2 tablespoons Parmesan cheese, shredded
- 1 teaspoon cream cheese, softened
- 1 small jalapeño pepper, chopped
- 1/8 teaspoon onion powder
- 1/8 teaspoon garlic powder

Directions:

1. Preheat a mini waffle iron and then grease it.
2. In a medium bowl, place all ingredients and mix until well combined.
3. Place half of the mixture into preheated waffle iron and cook for about 4-5 minutes or until golden brown.
4. Repeat with the remaining mixture.
5. Serve warm.

Nutrition: Calories: 170Net Carb: 0.9gFat: 9.9gSaturated Fat: 5.2gCarbohydrates: 0.1gDietary Fiber: 2. Sugar: 0.5gProtein: 8.6g

CONCLUSION

The most well-documented advantage of the keto diet is the rapid weight loss. Contrary to beliefs, many people describe a reduction in hunger. Not only that, ketones can also minimize acne, and even enhance cardioprotection and maintain nerve activity, either way, once you start buying avocado crates, especially if you have avocado crates problem , You can contact the doctor for their opinions and guidelines. obesity. Everyone's requirements are different, and they don't apply to you. This applies to most citizens. In addition to focusing on fat quality, you can also evaluate protein when choosing foods. In a keto diet, you only need moderate amounts of protein-about 20% of total calorie consumption can come from protein-and some nuts seem to be rich in protein.

From the perspective of minerals and vitamins, make sure to integrate fibrous fruits and vegetables (such as cabbage, broccoli, and cauliflower).

According to the person's situation, it takes about 2-4 days to enter ketosis (it is recommended that the carbohydrate is low enough). Likewise, the amount of carbohydrates required to achieve ketosis may vary from person to person. "The initial weight loss will be very rapid, but remember that most of it will be contained in glycogen (carbohydrates) and water. Later, due to insufficient calories and consumption of more fat as fuel, slow weight loss will follow. Come." As the expression develops, winning the game slowly and steadily is extremely effective for diet. You can easily lose weight with ketones, but you may need to stay vigilant for a long time to help your body adapt to new eating habits.

There is no doubt that chaff dominates in the low-carb world: they are awesome. For unlimited combinations of flavoring, sweetness or saltiness, you can add and change with very simple ingredients (only cheese and eggs). Use it alone or as a resource for seasonings and toppings. A simple calculation method is 1/2 cup 1 egg cheese per egg shell. Start adding coconut or almond flour. Check the cheese. Muffins can be frozen and processed, so a large portion can be made and stored for fast and extremely fast meals. If you don't have a waffle maker, just cook the mixture in a frying pan like pancakes and even cool it in a frying pan. They won't get all the fluffy aspects like using a waffle maker, but they will definitely be delicious.

Chaffle is a very mature and popular technology that can fix people on ships. Compared to most forms of keto bread, this crusty bread is more durable and better. "You may want a high-carbohydrate diet. A nonstick waffle maker can make life easier, and it's a compromise choice, and it's nice to embrace our happiness.

In summary, if you are very diligent and aware of this, a keto diet is healthy and helpful for your health and weight loss. The best way to monitor your commitment to ketones is to use a diet tracking app, where you can easily set the target amount of macronutrients/macrolysis (on ketones, fat is definitely 75% and carbohydrates is 5%, Protein is 20%) and check the label of the food you choose to eat.

For everything transitioning to a lifestyle, please give yourself some time to adapt. You can see some rapid changes almost immediately, but to reduce the burden, even if the rate of improvement slows down, you must follow the plan. Slowing down does not mean that the new diet has stopped working. This simply means that the body is actually adjusting itself to adapt to the new eating habits. Losing weight or reducing unnecessary excess weight is just a side effect of a healthy and better lifestyle that can support you in the long term (not only in the short term).

Lightning Source UK Ltd.
Milton Keynes UK
UKHW022010030521
383075UK00003B/264